FRUIT INFUSED

Contents

What will you find included in the ultimate Fruit Infused Water Book?

• One Fruit Infused Water recipe to cook every day of your life.
• A detailed list of what ingredients you will need to make your Fruit Infused Ware Recipes.
• A step by step guide on how to create your Fruit Infused Ware Recipes.
• A wide variety of drinks to satisfy all tastes and preferences.

Impress family and Friends: The Fruit Infused Water Recipes Cookbook has arrived!

So here you are! Ready to cook delicious Fruit Infused Water Recipes! Do you want to impress your family, friends or even give yourself a treat? Whether you are new to this or an experienced cook, here you will find all the tools you need to prepare exceptional dishes.

Now imagine being at home: You are working, doing your chores or coming back home after running you errands: All your looking for, craving for is a refreshing Fruit Infused Water Recipe....

Mango Fresca with Lime Juice

INGREDIENTS
- 1 tablespoon freshly squeezed Lime Juice
- 2 tablespoons Turbinado Sugar
- 3 cups filtered water
- 3 cup Mango pieces

PREPARATION
1. Add all ingredients to a blender.
2. Blend until liquefied.
3. Garnish with a slice of lime.
4. Serve over lots of ice.

Lime Fresca with Coconut Water and Watermelon

INGREDIENTS

- 3 cups coconut water
- 1 tablespoon freshly squeezed lime juice
- 2 seedless watermelon

PREPARATION

1. Puree the watermelon in a blender.
2. Place a fine-mesh sieve over a pitcher.
3. Pour the pureed watermelon through the sieve.
4. Discard pulp.
5. Stir in coconut water and lime juice.
6. Chill covered until cold.
7. Serve over ice.

Raspberry Fresca with Melon and Lime

INGREDIENTS

- 1 cup baking sugar
- 4 limes
- 2 cup raspberries
- 2 ripe honeydew melon

PREPARATION

1. Cut the melon in half.
2. Remove seeds with a spoon.
3. Cut flesh from peel and cut into chunks.
4. Place half of the melon in a large blender.
5. Process until liquefied.
6. Pour the liquefied melon into a fine mesh.
7. Sieve set over a large bowl.
8. Press the melon into the sieve.
9. Allow the juice to squeeze through into the bowl.
10. Scrape the flesh off of the sieve.
11. Repeat with remaining melon.
12. Transfer melon juice to a large pitcher.
13. Add four cups of water.
14. Combine lime juice and sugar in a bowl.
15. Stir until sugar is dissolved.
16. Pour the lime-sugar mixture into the pitcher.
17. Stir well.
18. Garnish with raspberries.
19. Serve over ice.

Cucumber Fresca with Kiwis and Cucumber

INGREDIENTS

- 3 packets Splenda
- 4 cups water
- Extra kiwi slices
- 8 kiwis
- 2 large cucumber

PREPARATION

1. Move the kiwi, cucumber, Splenda and water in a blender.
2. Puree until smooth for about 3-5 minutes.
3. Transfer to a pitcher.
4. Stir in the remaining water.

Mint Fresca with Honey and Lime Juice

INGREDIENTS
- 3 Tbsp. fresh mint leaves
- 1 tsp salt
- sparkling water
- mint sprigs for garnish
- 1 c water
- 1 c honey
- 3 c cantaloupe
- 1/3 c fresh lime juice

PREPARATION
1. Combine the honey and water in a small saucepan.
2. Heat over medium low heat until water and honey are combined.
3. Boil about 3-5 minutes.
4. Remove from heat and cool.
5. Combine honey syrup, cantaloupe, lime juice, mint leaves, and salt in a blender.
6. Puree until smooth.
7. Strain the cantaloupe mixture into another container.
8. Discard solids.
9. Pour cantaloupe juice over ice.
10. Fill the rest with sparkling water.
11. Mix equal parts cantaloupe juice and sparkling water in a pitcher.
12. Pour into glasses.
13. Garnish with a mint sprig and enjoy!

Lavender Water with Blueberries and Edible

INGREDIENTS

- Edible Flowers
- 48 ounces Water
- 1/4 pint Blueberries

PREPARATION

1. Add Fruits and edible flowers to a pitcher of water.
2. Cover and chill for 20-30 minutes.
3. Strain and add ice.
4. Pour into glasses and serve.

Infused Water with Mint and Strawberries

INGREDIENTS

- 1/2 cup fresh mint leaves
- Ice cubes
- Water
- 2 cup sliced strawberries
- 3 cup sliced cucumbers
- 1 limes

PREPARATION

1. Layer the strawberries, cucumbers, lime slices, and mint leaves in a pitcher with ice cubes.
2. Fill pitcher with water.
3. Chill for 10-15 minutes.
4. Serve and enjoy!

Detox Water with Oranges and Fresh Mint

INGREDIENTS

- 2 lemons
- 1/3 large cucumber
- 2 handful of fresh mint
- 3 liters' water
- 3 large oranges

PREPARATION

1. Put oranges, lemon and cucumber in water pitcher.
2. Mash fruits.
3. Take the mint.
4. Gently mash to release the natural oils.
5. Add to the pitcher.

Infused Water with Lemon, Mint and Blueberries

INGREDIENTS

- citrus cucumber
- apples, honeydew, blueberries
- Rosemary, basil, mint
- raspberry lemon
- watermelon mint
- tropical

PREPARATION

1. Add desired fruits to a pitcher.
2. Fill with water.
3. Allow fruit to soak for 5-8 hours in the fridge.
4. Add little more fruit.
5. Add more fruit for more flavor and sweetness.
6. Serve and enjoy.

Orange Water with Ice and Blueberries

INGREDIENTS

- 1 handful of blueberries
- ice
- 4 cups water
- 3 mandarin oranges

PREPARATION

1. Combine all ingredients in a pitcher.
2. Put in the fridge for 18-24 hours.
3. Squeeze in the juice of one mandarin orange.
4. Muddle the blueberries.
5. Serve cold.

Flavored Water with Strawberries, Lemon and Basil

INGREDIENTS

- 1 handful of basil
- Ice and cold filtered water
- 5 strawberries
- 1 lemon

PREPARATION

1. Fill juice pitcher to the top with ice and fruit.
2. Scrunch up the basil.
3. Cover with cold filtered water.
4. Infuse the water for 1-3 hours.
5. Poke a few holes in fruit with a fork.

Coconut Water with Peaches and Blackberries

INGREDIENTS

- 4 cups spring water
- 3 cups unsweetened coconut water
- 2-gallon clean glass jar
- 2 cup organic blueberries
- 1/2 cup organic blackberries
- 1 doughnut peaches

PREPARATION

1. Place blueberries and blackberries into the bottom of a jar.
2. Now the peach slices on top.
3. Pour the spring water and coconut water into the jar.
4. Stir the water.
5. Cover with a lid.
6. Put water into the refrigerator for 1-2 hours.
7. Drink within 2-3 days.

Kiwi Cold Cocktail with Filtered Water

INGREDIENTS

- 3 quarts filtered
- 4 ripe kiwis

PREPARATION

1. Add the sliced kiwis to a Mason jar.
2. Add the filtered water.
3. Refrigerate until cold and enjoy!

Cucumber Water with Strawberry and Ice

INGREDIENTS

- 4 slices of cucumber
- Ice
- Water
- 2 basil leaves
- 2 strawberry sliced

PREPARATION

1. Combine all the ingredients in a large glass.
2. Let sit for at least 5-7 minutes before serving.

Lemon with Raspberries and Spring Water

INGREDIENTS

- 2 large organic lemon
- 1 dried Medjool dates
- 2-gallon clean glass jar
- 3 cups organic raspberries
- 6 cups spring water

PREPARATION

1. Place raspberries into the bottom of a jar.
2. Add the dates.
3. Layer the lemon slices on top.
4. Pour water into jar and place lid on top.
5. Place water into the refrigerator.
6. Let infuse for 1-2 hours.

Melon with Watermelon and Filtered Water

INGREDIENTS

- 2 cup honeydew pieces
- 1 quarts filtered
- 2 cup cantaloupe pieces
- 3 cup watermelon pieces

PREPARATION

1. Move melons to a Mason jar.
2. Pour the water over top and chill.
3. Serve over ice.

Mint Drinks with Strawberries and Oranges

INGREDIENTS

- 1/4 orange
- 12 ounces filtered water
- 1/3 cup fresh mint
- 1 cup strawberries

PREPARATION

1. Move all fruits and herbs into the mason jar.
2. Fill to top with water.
3. Seal mason jar tightly.
4. Refrigerate overnight.

Ginger Water with Pineapple

INGREDIENTS

- piece ginger
- 3 quarts filtered
- 2 cup fresh pineapple pieces

PREPARATION

1. Move the pineapple and ginger to a Mason jar.
2. Pour water over top.
3. Refrigerate until cold.
4. Serve over ice and enjoy!

Lavender Mixer with Cucumber Water

INGREDIENTS
- 1/2 teaspoon dried culinary lavender
- 3 quarts filtered
- 2 cucumber

PREPARATION
1. Place the cucumbers and lavender to a Mason jar.
2. Add the filtered water.
3. Strain before serving.
4. Refrigerate until cold and enjoy!

Detox Water with Lemon and Grapefruit

INGREDIENTS

- 2 Cucumber
- 1 Fresh Mint
- Ice
- Water
- 1 Lemon
- 2 Lime
- 3 Grapefruit

PREPARATION

1. Combine water and ice in a glass.
2. Add lemon, lime, grapefruit, cucumber and mint.
3. Use slices of lemon, slice of grapefruit, slices of lime, slices of cucumber and mint leaves.
4. Stir and wait for 5-8 minutes.

Detox Water with Cucumber, Lemon and Grapefruit

INGREDIENTS

- 1/6 cucumber
- 3 mint leaves
- 1 lemon
- 1 lime
- 1-gallon spring water
- 1/3 grapefruit

PREPARATION

1. Combine all ingredients in a pitcher.
2. Refrigerate them for 2-3 hours before serving.
3. Drink throughout the day.

Detox Drink with Lemon and Ginger Root

INGREDIENTS

- Juice of 1/3 lemon
- 1-inch knob of ginger root
- 2-ounce glass water

PREPARATION

1. Put the lemon juice to a glass.
2. Finely grate the ginger.
3. Add to the glass of water.

Orange Water with Blueberries and Ice

INGREDIENTS
- 1 handful of blueberries
- ice
- 4 cups water
- 3 mandarin oranges

PREPARATION
1. Combine all ingredients in a pitcher.
2. Put in the fridge for all day long.
3. Allow the water to infuse.
4. Squeeze in the juice of one mandarin orange.
5. Muddle the blueberries.
6. Serve cold.

Mint Water with Lemon and Ice

INGREDIENTS
- sprigs of mint
- ice
- 4 cups water
- 1 lemon

PREPARATION
1. Combine all ingredients in a pitcher.
2. Put in the fridge for 2-3 hours.
3. Allow the water to infuse.
4. Squeeze in the juice of lemon.
5. Serve cold.

Healthy Detox Water with Watermelon

INGREDIENTS

- 2 cups Water
- 3 cups Seedless Watermelon

PREPARATION

1. Place Watermelon in pitcher.
2. Cover with Water.
3. Keep them in the refrigerator for few hours before drinking.

Mint Water with Raspberries and Lime

INGREDIENTS

- 1 Tablespoons raspberries
- 3 tablespoons fresh mint leaves
- 2 lime
- 3 liters cold spring water

PREPARATION

1. Microwave for 20-30 seconds.
2. Cool and slice then.
3. Place raspberries, mint, lime and water in a large jug.
4. Stir and serve.

Spa Water with Cucumber, Lemon and Mint

INGREDIENTS
- 2 Lemon
- 8 Mint Leaves
- 6 C. Water
- 2 Cucumber

PREPARATION
1. Combine all ingredients in an airtight container.
2. Leave overnight in the fridge.

Detox Drink with Cider Vinegar and Cinnamon

INGREDIENTS

- 1/2 Teaspoon Cinnamon
- 1/3 Teaspoon sweetener
- Half of an apple
- 6 oz. of Water
- 3 Tablespoon Apple Cider Vinegar
- 2 Tablespoon fresh Lemon Juice

PREPARATION

1. Combine all the ingredients except apples in a blender.
2. Blend for about 10-15 seconds.
3. Add slices of Apple.
4. Drink and then eat the apple slices.

Herb Water with Pineapple and Thyme Ice

INGREDIENTS

- a sprig of mint, basil, sage, rosemary, tarragon and thyme
- water
- ice
- 2 cups berries, citrus, melons, pineapple

PREPARATION

1. Add a sprig of fresh herbs to jar.
2. Press and twist with muddler.
3. Don't pulverize the herbs into bits.
4. Add fruit to jar and press.
5. Twist with muddler.
6. Fill jar with ice cubes.
7. Add water to top of jar.
8. Cover and refrigerate for up to 2-3 days.

Cucumber Water with Lemon and Orange

INGREDIENTS

- 2 large orange
- 2 large cucumber
- 3 half-gallon of water
- 2 large lemon
- 3 large lime

PREPARATION

1. Place all the sliced fruits and the cucumber in a glass pitcher.
2. Add water.
3. Refrigerate for 2-3 hours.
4. Serve in glasses over ice.

Cucumber Water with Lemon and Fresh Mint

INGREDIENTS

- 1 lemon slices
- 3 sprigs of fresh mint
- 2 sprigs of rosemary
- 3 cups water
- 8 thin slices of cucumber

PREPARATION

1. Put water in pitcher.
2. Add lemon and cucumber slices.
3. Crush mint and rosemary.
4. Add to other ingredients.
5. Refrigerate for 3-5 hours.
6. Serve over ice in tall glasses.
7. Garnish with a lemon wedge.

Melon Water with Cucumber and Cantaloupe

INGREDIENTS

- 1/3 honeydew melon
- 1/2 cantaloupe
- 2 half-gallon water
- 2 large cucumbers

PREPARATION

1. Place cucumber and melons in a glass pitcher.
2. Add water and refrigerate for 2-4 hours.
3. Serve over ice garnishing with melon balls.

Lime Water with Honeydew Melon and Mint

INGREDIENTS
- 2 lime
- 3 sprigs of mint
- 1 gallon of water
- 3 slices honeydew melon

PREPARATION
1. Add melon slices, lime slices and mint sprigs to a large pitcher.
2. Fill with half-gallon of water.
3. Refrigerate 3-5 hours.
4. Serve in ice-filled glasses.

Berry Water with Rosemary

INGREDIENTS

- 3 inch sprigs of fresh rosemary
- 2 half-gallon of water
- 2 cup fresh blueberries

PREPARATION

1. Add blueberries and rosemary sprigs to a large pitcher.
2. Fill with the half-gallon of water.
3. Refrigerate 3-4 hours.
4. Serve in ice-filled glasses and enjoy!

Lemon Water with Lavender

INGREDIENTS

- 1/3 cup fresh lavender
- 1 gallon of water
- 2 large lemons

PREPARATION

1. Add lemon slices and lavender to pitcher.
2. Pour water over both.
3. Refrigerate for 3-5 hours.
4. Serve over ice garnishing with a sprig of lavender.

Basil Water with Lemon and Fresh Mint

INGREDIENTS

- 8 cups water
- 4 cups ice cubes
- Fresh mint
- 3 lemons
- 2 cups firmly packed fresh mint

PREPARATION

1. Place lemon slices in a large pitcher.
2. Rub the mint to bruise the leaves slightly.
3. Add to the pitcher with lemon.
4. Pour in the water.
5. Cover and sit for 5-7 hours.
6. Strain lemon and water mixture.
7. Discard herbs.
8. Divide lemon slices and additional fresh mint among 5-7 glasses.
9. Add ice cubes in each glasses.
10. Fill with lemon water.

Orange Water with Lime and Cilantro Leaves

INGREDIENTS

- 3 large orange
- 1/2 cup cilantro leaves
- 1 gallon of water
- 2 large lemons
- 2 large lime

PREPARATION

1. Add citrus slices to a pitcher.
2. Fill with the half-gallon of water and refrigerate for 3-5 hours.
3. Serve in ice-filled glasses.
4. Garnish with citrus slice.

Fruit Water with Apple Chunks

INGREDIENTS

- 1 gallon of water
- 3 cups frozen apple chunks

PREPARATION

1. Add frozen fruit to a pitcher.
2. Pour water over fruit and refrigerate for 20-30 minutes.
3. Stir to distribute fruit flavor.
4. Serve in glasses with ice cubes.

Fresh Mint Water with Oranges

INGREDIENTS
- 8 mint leaves
- 1 gallon of water
- 4 large oranges

PREPARATION
1. Put sliced oranges and mint leaves in pitcher.
2. Add water and refrigerate for 3-5 hours.
3. Pour over ice.
4. Garnish with a sprig of mint and orange slice.

Healthy Basil Water with Watermelon

INGREDIENTS
- 8 basil leaves
- 1 gallon of water
- 3 cups seedless watermelon

PREPARATION
1. Pour water over melon and basil.
2. Refrigerate for about 3-5 hours.
3. Serve over ice garnished with sprig of basil.

Fruit Water with Apples, Strawberries and Raspberries

INGREDIENTS

- 1 Handful of raspberries
- 1 Handful of mint leaves
- 1 gallon of water
- 2 each apple, lemon, orange, pear
- 3 large strawberries

PREPARATION

1. Cut large slices of each fruit.
2. Place them in a glass pitcher.
3. Add cold water.
4. Refrigerate for 3-5 hours.
5. Serve over ice in tall glasses.

Lavender Water with Blueberries and Edible

INGREDIENTS

- Edible Flowers
- 48 ounces Water
- 1/3 pint Blueberries

PREPARATION

1. Add Fruits and edible flowers to a pitcher.
2. Cover and wait for about 20-30 minutes.
3. Strain and add ice.
4. Pour into tall glasses and serve.

Mint Infused Water with Cucumber and Ice

INGREDIENTS
- 1/2 cup fresh mint leaves
- Ice cubes
- Water
- 2 cup sliced strawberries
- 3 cup sliced cucumbers
- 3 limes

PREPARATION
1. Layer the strawberries, cucumbers, lime slices, and mint leaves in a pitcher with ice cubes.
2. Fill pitcher with water.
3. Wait for 10-15 minutes and serve.

Detox Water with Oranges and Fresh Mint

INGREDIENTS

- 2 lemons
- 1 large cucumber
- 1 handful of fresh mint
- 3 liters' water
- 3 large oranges

PREPARATION

1. Put oranges, lemon and cucumber in a pitcher.
2. Mash the fruits.
3. Take the mint and gently mash.
4. Now add them to the pitcher.
5. Add water to the pitcher.
6. Stir to begin the infusion process.
7. Drink immediately.

Strawberry Water with Lemon and Basil

INGREDIENTS
- Ice and cold filtered water
- 3 slices of watermelon
- Small handful of basil
- Ice and cold filtered water
- 6 strawberries
- 1 lemon
- 1 Small handful of basil

PREPARATION
1. Fill juice pitcher to the top with ice and fruit.
2. Slightly scrunch up the basil.
3. Cover with cold filtered water.
4. Poke a few holes in fruits for instant flavor.

Flavored Detox Water with Strawberries

INGREDIENTS

- 4 slices of watermelon
- 1 Small handful of basil
- Ice and cold filtered water
- 5 strawberries
- 1/4 lemon
- 1 Small handful of basil
- Ice and cold filtered water

PREPARATION

1. Fill juice pitcher to the top with ice and fruit.
2. Slightly scrunch up the basil.
3. Cover with cold filtered water.

Detox Green Tea with Honey and Lemon

INGREDIENTS

- 1/2 tsp honey
- 1 strawberry
- 3 slices cucumber
- 2 green tea bag
- 3 slice lemon

PREPARATION

1. Brew 5-7 fluid ounces of water to make green tea.
2. Keep green tea in refrigerator for 5-8 minutes.
3. Add cucumber, lemon, strawberries and honey.
4. Stir to mix ingredients.
5. Add ice.
6. Drink daily as a natural detox.

Detox Water with Strawberry, Cucumber and Ice

INGREDIENTS

- 2 strawberry sliced
- 4 slices of cucumber
- Ice
- Water
- 2 Basil leaves

PREPARATION

1. Combine all the ingredients in a glass.
2. Wait for about 5-8 minutes.
3. Serve and Enjoy!

Spa Water with Blueberries and Lemon

INGREDIENTS
- 1/4 cup raspberries
- 2 lemon
- 2 cups water
- 1/3 cup blueberries

PREPARATION
1. Add all ingredients to a large glass.
2. Cover with lid and allow to chill overnight in the refrigerator.
3. Drink throughout the day.

Spa Water with Cinnamon and Apple Slice

INGREDIENTS
- 3 Cinnamon Stick
- 2 Apple thinly sliced

PREPARATION
1. Drop apple slices in the bottom of a pitcher.
2. Now the cinnamon stick.
3. Cover with ice and water.
4. Keep in the fridge for 1-3 hours before serving.

Detox Water with Raspberry and Orange

INGREDIENTS

- 3 oranges
- 1 quart's water
- 3 cups fresh raspberries

PREPARATION

1. Add raspberries to a jar.
2. Break up gently with a wooden spoon.
3. Cut the oranges into wedges.
4. Squeeze juice into the jar.
5. Toss the wedges in too.
6. Add water.
7. Cover and chill until ready to serve.

Rose Water with Mint Sprigs

INGREDIENTS

- 1/3 tsp rose water
- 1 quart's water
- 3 mint sprigs

PREPARATION

1. Put mint sprigs and rose water to a jar.
2. Add water and rose water.
3. Cover and chill until ready to serve.

Rosemary Water with Cubed Watermelon

INGREDIENTS

- 2 sprig rosemary
- 1 quart's water
- 3 cups cubed watermelon

PREPARATION

1. Put rosemary in a jar.
2. Massage gently.
3. Add watermelon to jar and gently mash.
4. Pour in water.
5. Cover and chill until ready to serve.

Spa Water with Ice and Strawberry

INGREDIENTS

- 2 pitcher filtered water
- ice
- 2 lb. strawberries

PREPARATION

1. Add strawberries and water to a pitcher.
2. Cover and refrigerate for about 4-6 hours.
3. Add ice before serving.

Infused Water with Fruit, Mint Leaves and Ice

INGREDIENTS

- 1/3 cup fruit
- 1/2 cup ice
- 1 mint leaves
- 12 oz. mason jar
- 2 cup water

PREPARATION

1. Move fruit in the bottom of jar.
2. Pour water in.
3. Stir fruit around.
4. Press on the fruit lightly.
5. Add mint leaves.
6. Refrigerate for about 1-3 hours.
7. Add ice just before serving.

Detox Drink with Pineapple and Apple Cider Vinegar

INGREDIENTS
- 1/3 Cup Pineapple
- 2 teaspoons Apple Cider Vinegar
- 6 Medium Basil leafs
- 12 oz. Cold Water
- 1/3 Cup Ice
- 6 Strawberries

PREPARATION
1. Fill cup with water and ice.
2. Add the apple cider vinegar.
3. Add all fruit to the cold water.
4. Smash and squeeze into the drink.
5. Add the basil leafs and stir.
6. Wait for about 20-30 minutes before drinking.
7. Drink and enjoy!

Detox Water with Pineapple and Strawberries

INGREDIENTS
- 1/3 Cup Pineapple
- 1/2 teaspoons Apple Cider Vinegar
- 3 Medium Basil leafs
- 12 oz. Cold Water
- 1 Cup Ice
- 4 Strawberries

PREPARATION
1. Fill cup with water and ice.
2. Add the apple cider vinegar.
3. Add all fruit to the cold water and smash.
4. Squeeze into the drink.
5. Add the basil leafs and stir.
6. Wait for about 20-30 minutes before drinking.

Detox Drink with Lime and Green Tea

INGREDIENTS

- 3 Green Tea Bag
- 1 Cup of Mint Leaves
- Water
- 2 Lime

PREPARATION

1. Fill a large mason jar.
2. Add tea bag.
3. Keep in fridge for about 25-30 minutes.
4. Cut up lime and chop up mint.
5. Place in the water.
6. Cover and take out tea bag.
7. Keep in the fridge for about 25-30 more minutes.
8. Serve and Enjoy!

Kiwi Water with Strawberries

INGREDIENTS

- 3 kiwis
- 5 strawberries
- 1-gallon cold water

PREPARATION

1. Mix all ingredients together.
2. Keep them in the refrigerator for 2-3 hours before serving.
3. Discard after 1-2 days.

Metabolism Water with Apple and Cinnamon

INGREDIENTS
- 5 Apples
- 4 Cinnamon Sticks
- 1 Gallon Water

PREPARATION
1. Simmer One Gallon of Water on the stove.
2. Core apples and place in the pot of water.
3. Add Cinnamon Sticks.
4. Simmer for about 10-15 minutes.
5. Add Apple Cinnamon and water into a glass pitcher.
6. Refrigerate for about 2-3 hours.
7. Add additional water.

Cucumber Lime with Mint and Lemon

INGREDIENTS

Strawberry-Lemon with Basil
- 1/3 cup sliced strawberries
- 1/4 lemon
- 1 cup fresh basil leaves
- 1/3 cucumber
- 1 lime
- 1/3 cup fresh mint leaves

Watermelon Mint
- 1 cup fresh mint leaves
- 2 cup cubed watermelon

Pineapple-Orange with Ginger
- 1/4 orange, sliced
- 2 tablespoons freshly grated ginger
- 1 cup cubed pineapple

PREPARATION
1. Gather all the ingredients together.
2. Place fruit and herbs in the bottom of a jar.
3. Muddle with a wooden spoon.
4. Fill jar with water and give it a taste.
5. Add some agave and mix until dissolved.
6. Refrigerate overnight for maximum flavor.

Detox Drink with Lemon and Lime Water

INGREDIENTS

- ice cubes
- water
- 2 lemon
- 2 lime

PREPARATION

1. Slice the lemon and lime.
2. Add to a pitcher.
3. Top with water and pop in a fridge.
4. Add ice and serve!

Infused Water with Raspberries and Blueberries

INGREDIENTS

- 1/3 cup of fresh blueberries
- 1 cup of fresh raspberries
- 6 oz. canning jar

PREPARATION

1. Add the fresh blueberries and raspberries.
2. Gently mash the fruit down with a fork.
3. Fill the jar with water.
4. Place the cover on.
5. Shake once and place in the fridge overnight.
6. Refrigerate for overnight.

Detox Water with Orange, Lemon, Lime and Ginger

INGREDIENTS

- 2 slices fresh ginger
- 18 mint leaves
- 5 cups ice
- Water
- 2 orange
- 3 lime
- 2 lemon
- 1/3 cucumber

PREPARATION

1. Slice the fruit and cucumbers.
2. Fill a large container dispenser layering ice and the ingredients.
3. Top with cold water.
4. Wait for about 30-45 minutes.
5. Serve and Enjoy!

Fruit Water with Herb Flavor and Ice

INGREDIENTS

- a sprig of mint, basil, sage, rosemary
- water
- ice
- 1 cups berries, citrus, melons, pineapple

PREPARATION

1. Add a sprig of fresh herbs to jar.
2. Press and twist with muddler.
3. Add fruit to jar, press and twist with muddler.
4. Fill jar with ice cubes.
5. Add water to top of jar.
6. Cover and refrigerate for up to 1-3 days.

Healthy Drinks with Strawberries and Lemons

INGREDIENTS
- 1 Handful ripe raspberries
- 3 sliced lemons
- 6 sliced strawberries

PREPARATION
1. Slice all ingredients.
2. Put into a jar.
3. Fill glass with water.
4. Place in the refrigerator overnight.
5. Enjoy in the sunshine!

Detox Drink with Cucumber, Ginger and Fresh Mint

INGREDIENTS

- 2 Cucumber
- 3 Tablespoon grated Fresh Ginger
- 2 Lime
- Fresh Mint
- 3 quarts' water
- 2 Lemon

PREPARATION

1. Cut the lemon, lime and cucumber into thin slices.
2. Grate the ginger.
3. Combine all of ingredients and stir.
4. Place the detox water in the fridge for 3-5 hours.

Fat Flush with Lemon and Blueberries

INGREDIENTS

- 1/3 cup raspberries
- 2 lemon
- 2 cups water
- 1 cup blueberries

PREPARATION

1. Add all ingredients to a large glass.
2. Cover with lid and chill overnight in the refrigerator.
3. Drink throughout the day.

Infused Water with Lime, Fresh Cilantro and Watermelon

INGREDIENTS

- 2 lime
- 4 sprigs of fresh cilantro
- 2 heaping cup of watermelon
- 3 cups filtered water
- 16 ice cubes

PREPARATION

1. Combine all of the ingredients in a large carafe.
2. Refrigerate for about 8-10 hours.
3. Drink within 1-2 days.

Infused Water with Granny Smith Apples and Lemongrass

INGREDIENTS

- 1 large Granny Smith apple
- 4 quarter size coins of peeled ginger
- 3 stalks of lemongrass
- 3 cups filtered water
- 12 ice cubes

PREPARATION

1. Combine all the ingredients in a large carafe.
2. Refrigerate for about 10-12 hours.

Infused Water with Basil, Cucumber and Lime

INGREDIENTS
- 3 medium lemon
- 2 medium lime
- 1 cup of fresh basil
- 24 oz. canning jar
- 2 medium cucumber

PREPARATION
1. Add the cucumber sliced fruit and basil to the canning jar.
2. Mash them down a bit.
3. Fill the jar with water and let refrigerate overnight.
4. Enjoy ice cold!

Detox Drink with Mint, Lemon and Watermelon

INGREDIENTS

- 6 Mint leaves
- 1/3 lemon cut into slices
- 1 Cup Watermelon Cut into chunks

PREPARATION

1. Fill a glass with ice and cold water.
2. Add watermelon, mint and melon to water.
3. Wait for about 25-30 minutes.
4. Drink and Enjoy!

Detox Drink with Lime, Mint Leaves and Ice

INGREDIENTS

- 2 lemon or lime
- 1 handful of fresh mint leaves
- Ice cubes
- 3 liters of water
- 1 watermelon

PREPARATION

1. Slice up a good amount of watermelon into cubes.
2. Rind and put them into a jug.
3. Cut lime into wedges and toss with the watermelon.
4. Add a handful of fresh, fragrant, mint leaves.
5. Pour in cool water.
6. Fill the jug to the top.
7. Wait overnight in the fridge.
8. Put in a generous of ice cubes.
9. Pour and enjoy daily.

Spa Water with Strawberries, Lemon and Herbs

INGREDIENTS

- 2 small cucumber
- 4 medium sized strawberries
- 2 small sprigs of fresh herbs
- 2 gallon of water
- 3 large lemon thinly sliced

PREPARATION

1. Place all the sliced fruits and veggies into a pitcher.
2. Add the sprigs of herbs.
3. Fill the pitcher with water.
4. Refrigerate for about 5-7 hours.

Dream Water and Pitcher with Cilantro

INGREDIENTS

- 2 small bunch cilantro
- 2 small bunch Italian parsley
- 1 handful of frozen cranberries
- 1 large pitcher
- 2 lemon thinly sliced
- 1 cucumber thinly sliced

PREPARATION

1. Mix all ingredients together and refrigerate.
2. Continue to refill with water throughout the day.

Detox Juice with Pears, Carrots and Lemon

INGREDIENTS

- 2 lemon
- 3 cups honeydew melon cubed
- 2 orange
- 2-inch piece ginger
- 3 pears
- 3 carrots
- 1 stalks celery
- 3 nectarines

PREPARATION

1. Juice all the ingredients.
2. Drink the green juice within 18-24 hours.

Strawberry Water with Basil, Watermelon and Lemon

INGREDIENTS
- 3 slices of watermelon
- 1 Small handful of basil
- Ice and cold filtered water
- 5 strawberries
- 1 lemon
- 1 Small handful of basil
- Ice and cold filtered water

PREPARATION
1. Fill juice pitcher to the top with ice and fruit.
2. Slightly scrunch up the basil.
3. Cover with cold filtered water.
4. Infuse water for about 1-3 hours.

Herb Water with Pineapple, Berries and Mint

INGREDIENTS

- a sprig of mint, basil, sage
- water
- ice
- 2 cups berries, citrus, melons, pineapple

PREPARATION

1. Add a sprig of fresh herbs to jar.
2. Press and twist with muddler.
3. Add fruit to jar and press.
4. Twist with muddler.
5. Fill the jar with ice cubes.
6. Add water to top of jar.
7. Cover and refrigerate for 1-3 days.

Infused Water with Raspberry, Watermelon and Honeydew

INGREDIENTS
- 1 citrus cucumber
- 1 each apple, honeydew
- 1 each Rosemary, basil, mint
- 1 raspberry
- 2 watermelon mint
- 1 tropical

PREPARATION
1. Add desired fruits to a pitcher.
2. Fill with water.
3. Allow fruit to soak for about 3-5 hours in the fridge.
4. Serve and enjoy!

Infused Water with Mint, Strawberries and Lime

INGREDIENTS

- 1 limes
- 1 cup fresh mint leaves
- Ice cubes
- Water
- 2 cup sliced strawberries
- 3 cup sliced cucumbers

PREPARATION

1. Layer the strawberries, cucumbers, lime slices, and mint leaves with the ice cubes.
2. Fill jar with water.
3. Wait for about 8-10 minutes.
4. Serve and enjoy!

Detox Water with Lemon, Cucumber and Orange

INGREDIENTS

- 2 lemon
- 1 large cucumber
- 2 handful of fresh mint
- 3 liters' water
- 1 large orange

PREPARATION

1. Put oranges, lemon and cucumber in the water pitcher.
2. Gently mash fruits.
3. Take the mint and gently mash.
4. Add to the pitcher.
5. Add water to the pitcher.
6. Stir to begin the infusion process.
7. Drink immediately.

Detox Water with Organic Lemon and Cucumber

INGREDIENTS

- 1 cucumber sliced
- 8 mint leaves
- 2 gallon of water
- 3 whole organic lemon

PREPARATION

1. Wash and dry the lemon.
2. Slice and remove seeds.
3. Fill pitcher with distilled water.
4. Add lemons, cucumbers and mint.
5. Refrigerate for 10-12 hours and enjoy!

Vitamin Water with Blackberries, Glutamine and Cherries

INGREDIENTS
- 10 ml Glutamine Powder
- 1 Pinch Himalayan Crystal Salt
- 600 ml Filtered Alkaline Water
- 1/3 Pomegranate Seeds
- 1 Cup Blackberries
- 2 Cup Cherries

PREPARATION
1. Muddle blackberries, cherries and pomegranate in a bowl.
2. Add to glass.
3. Add remaining ingredients and stir.
4. Refrigerate for about 3-5 hours.

Natural Drink with Grapefruit, Lemon and Valencia Orange

INGREDIENTS

- 6 Kumquats
- 6 g Camu Camu Powder
- 1 Pinch Himalayan Crystal Salt
- 550ml Filtered Alkaline Water
- 1 Grapefruit squeezed Grapefruit Juice
- 1/4 Lemon
- 1/3 Lime
- 1/3 Valencia Orange

PREPARATION

1. Juice grapefruit.
2. Add to a large mason jar.
3. Add remaining ingredients and stir.
4. Refrigerate for 2-5 hours.

Detox Water with Watermelon, Strawberries and Rosemary

INGREDIENTS

- 4 g Vitamin B Complex Powder
- 4 drops Valarian Root Extract
- 1 Pinch Himalayan Crystal Salt
- 650ml Filtered Alkaline Water
- 3 Cups Watermelon
- 2 Cup Strawberries
- 3 Sprigs Rosemary

PREPARATION

1. Muddle strawberries and rosemary in a bowl.
2. Add to a large mason jar and add remaining ingredients.
3. Stir and refrigerate for about 3-5 hours.

Dried Lemongrass with Fresh Mint and Pineapple

INGREDIENTS

- 3 Lychees
- 2" Fresh Dried Lemongrass
- 3 g Scoop Probiotics
- 2 Pinch Himalayan Crystal Salt
- 650ml Filtered Alkaline Water
- 2 Cup Pineapple
- 6 Sprigs Fresh Mint
- 2" Ginger

PREPARATION

1. Muddle lychees, ginger and mint in a small bowl.
2. Add to a large mason jar and add remaining ingredients.
3. Stir and refrigerate for 3-5 hours.

Orange Water with Blueberries and Ice

INGREDIENTS
- 1 handful of blueberries
- ice
- 5 cups water
- 3 mandarin oranges

PREPARATION
1. Combine all ingredients in a pitcher.
2. Put in the fridge for about 18-20 hours.
3. Squeeze in the juice of one mandarin orange.
4. Muddle the blueberries to intensify flavor a bit.
5. Serve cold.

Infused Water with Rosemary, Cucumber and Raspberry

INGREDIENTS

- 2 citrus cucumber
- 2 each apple, honeydew, cantaloupe
- 2 each Rosemary, basil, mint
- 2 raspberry
- 3 watermelon mint
- 1 tropical

PREPARATION

1. Add desired fruits to a pitcher.
2. Fill with water.
3. Allow fruit to soak for 3-5 hours in the fridge.
4. Serve and enjoy!

Detox Water with Orange, Lemon and Fresh Mint

INGREDIENTS
- 2 lemon
- 1 large cucumber
- 2 handful of fresh mint
- 3 liters' water
- 1 large orange

PREPARATION
1. Put oranges, lemon and cucumber in the water pitcher.
2. Gently mash fruits.
3. Take the mint and gently mash to release the natural oils.
4. Add to the pitcher.
5. Add water to the pitcher and stir.
6. Serve immediately.

Mint Infused Water with Lime, Cucumbers and Strawberries

INGREDIENTS

- 1 limes
- 1 cup fresh mint leaves
- Ice cubes
- Water
- 2 cup sliced strawberries
- 3 cup sliced cucumbers

PREPARATION

1. Layer the strawberries, cucumbers, lime slices, and mint leaves with the ice cubes.
2. Fill jar with water.
3. Wait for about 7-10 minutes.
4. Serve and enjoy!

Basil Infused Water with Lemon, Lime and Cucumber

INGREDIENTS

- 2 medium lemon
- 3 medium lime sliced
- 1 cup of fresh basil
- 24 oz. canning jar
- 2 medium cucumber

PREPARATION

1. Add the cucumber, sliced fruit and basil to the canning jar.
2. Mash them down a bit.
3. Fill the jar with water and refrigerate overnight.
4. Enjoy ice cold!

Infused Water with Mango and Basil

INGREDIENTS

- 1.1/2 handful fresh basil
- 3 quarts' water
- 1 mango

PREPARATION

1. Put all the ingredients in a carafe.
2. Refrigerate for about 1-3 hours.

Cucumber Water with Lemon and Ice

INGREDIENTS

- 1 cucumber
- Ice
- 2 liters' water
- 2 liters of fruit infused water
- 1/3 lemon to 1 lemon

PREPARATION

1. Add the lemon and cucumber to a jug.
2. Put water and ice on top.
3. Keep them for about 1-3 hours.

Apple Water with Cinnamon

INGREDIENTS

- 2 Thinly sliced apple
- 3 Cinnamon Stick
- 2 liters of fruit infused water

PREPARATION

1. Put the apple slices in a big jug.
2. Top it up with water and ice.

Detox Water with Orange and Ginger

INGREDIENTS

- 1 an orange
- 2 inch strip of ginger
- 2 liters of fruit infused water

PREPARATION

1. Add the peeled and sliced ginger in a jug.
2. Add orange slices.
3. Squeeze a few of the orange slices.
4. Top with water and keep them for 1-3 hours.

Infused Water with Mint and Peach

INGREDIENTS

- 10 peach slices
- Water
- 2 liters of fruit infused water
- 2 sprig of Mint

PREPARATION

1. Muddle a few mint leaves.
2. Add peaches and top with water.
3. Garnish with peaches and mint leaves.

Infused Water with Basil and Mango

INGREDIENTS

- 2 ripened mango
- 7 basil leaves
- 2 liters of fruit infused water

PREPARATION

1. Tear the basil leaves.
2. Add them along with the mango to a jug.
3. Top with water and ice.
4. Serve and enjoy!

Detox Water with Rosemary, Strawberries and Ice

INGREDIENTS

- **3 cups of ice**
- **Water**
- **4 sprigs rosemary**
- **12 strawberries quartered**

PREPARATION

1. Move the rosemary and strawberries in a pitcher.
2. Pour ice and water on top.
3. Keep them in the fridge for 1-3 hours before serving.
4. When the water is down refill again.
5. Place back in the fridge.
6. Store in the fridge up to 18-24 hours.

Infused Water with Orange, Pineapple and Ice

INGREDIENTS

- 1 cups of ice
- 2 orange
- Water
- 1 cup pineapple

PREPARATION

1. Add the orange and pineapple slices in a pitcher.
2. Top with ice and water.
3. Sit the pitcher in the fridge for 1-2 hours.
4. Refill with water when reduce and place back in the fridge.

Infused Water with Fresh Mint and Orange

INGREDIENTS

- 8 Strawberries
- 3 sprigs of fresh mint
- 2 Orange

PREPARATION

1. Add the orange and strawberries in a pitcher.
2. Squeeze and slightly twist the mint.
3. Do not tear apart.
4. Add the mint leaves to the fruit.
5. Pour ice and water on top.
6. Keep the pitcher in the fridge for 1-3 hours.
7. Refill with water when it is down.
8. Place back in the fridge.

Infused Water with Tangerine and Strawberries

INGREDIENTS

- 1 tangerine rind
- Water
- 1 cup strawberries

PREPARATION

1. Place the tangerine rind and strawberries into a teapot.
2. Cover with water and boil.
3. cover the nose of tea pot with a coffee filter and serve.

www.ingramcontent.com/pod-product-compliance
Lightning Source LLC
Chambersburg PA
CBHW071209280526
45787CB00002B/621